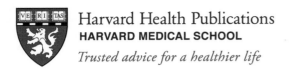

Harvard Health Publications
HARVARD MEDICAL SCHOOL
Trusted advice for a healthier life

Dear Reader,

You know core work is important. Still, you may be cautious about trying core exercises—perhaps because you've been unwell, you're afraid you'll hurt yourself, or you're concerned that you might exacerbate an existing injury. There are a lot of vigorous core exercise programs that may indeed cause problems if you dive in too quickly and attempt advanced moves when you're not ready for them.

That's why we've designed this program of gentle core exercises. It enables you to get started in a safe, easy way and progress at your own pace. While it incorporates much of the same basic information as our regular *Core Exercises* Special Health Report, this one provides gentler exercises, along with tips for tailoring the program to your needs. As we say, start low and go slow. That means taking your time and listening to your body. Do only as much as you can while maintaining good posture and alignment. Even if you do half the number of the exercises in one of our workouts, you'll be benefiting, because any exercise is better than none.

Our program also has a second group of people in mind—those who work at desk jobs and spend too much of the day sitting. You may not have enough time to go to the gym during lunch. But you can easily slip the simple, inconspicuous exercises in our Office Workout into your day.

If you are worried about injuring yourself, rest assured, most of these exercises are used in physical therapy, so they are very safe. If you have a health issue, however, get clearance from your doctor before trying them. And remember: if something hurts, don't do it. As you gain proficiency, then you can add more repetitions of exercises or move up to harder variations.

We hope your response to this report will be, "Yes, I can do this." As your core muscles get stronger, on-the-job tasks and everyday acts will become easier. So will pleasurable pursuits like golfing, tennis, biking, and quite possibly even sex. No less important, many of our exercises help your posture and improve balance, which makes debilitating falls less likely to happen at any age.

Here's our promise: No fancy exercise clothes. No pricey equipment. Just gains you'll begin to feel and see every day for a small investment of time.

Sincerely,

Edward Phillips, MD

Edward M. Phillips, M.D.
Medical Editor

Josie Gardiner

Josie Gardiner
Master Trainer

The importance of your core

Why spend time building up your core? Many people equate the core solely with rippling abdominal muscles. But the core reaches well beyond the abs, to muscles in your back, sides, pelvis, and buttocks that are essential to most of the movements you make. A surprising number of everyday actions—bending, twisting, and rotating your body, as well as standing upright—are ruled by your core. So whether you care about six-pack abs or just getting through the day more easily, it's worth paying attention to your core muscles.

Of course, many strenuous workouts enhance core strength. But not everyone is able to do those—

and frankly, some of them can cause injury if you don't do them properly. That's why we've compiled this program of gentle core exercises to complement our standard *Core Exercises* report—because people of all ages and fitness levels can benefit from core strengthening. Maybe you have an illness or injury that prevents heavy-duty core work. Maybe your age makes you reluctant to try some of the more challenging exercises. Maybe you have a desk job that keeps you sitting all day, but you have five minutes here and there to "work out at work." If any of these apply to you, these lighter core workouts may be exactly what you need. Gentle core work is much better than no core work at all.

Figure 1: Front and back core muscles

Your core is composed of many different muscles in the abdomen, back, sides, pelvis, and buttocks. These muscles work together to allow you to bend, twist, rotate, and stand upright.

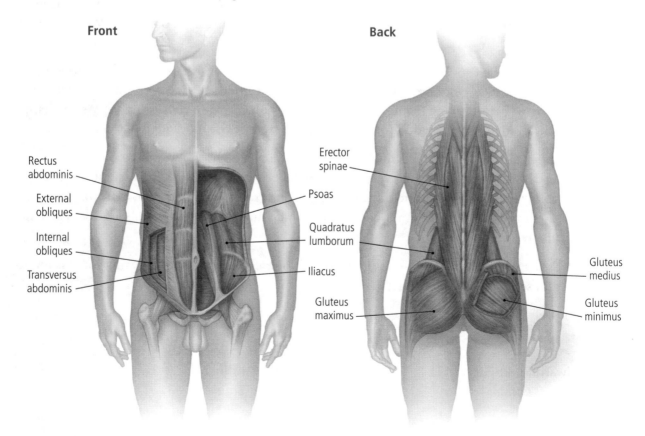

Got back pain?

Sadly, no magic cure is available for low back pain, a scourge that causes wincing and far worse in an estimated four out of five Americans at some point in their lives. Low back pain is the major reason cited for limited activity in adults, and it trails only respiratory infections in prompting visits to the doctor. And even though nearly half of people reporting low back pain feel better within a week, others may still be struggling with it a year or two later or have recurring episodes.

If you find yourself afflicted, call your doctor for advice. Muscle or bone conditions—a muscle spasm, perhaps, or osteoarthritis—are most often at fault, but back pain sometimes signals an illness, such as a urinary tract infection or appendicitis. What's more, notes the American Academy of Physical Medicine and Rehabilitation, ignoring back pain may compound it. Shifting your posture and gait to ease discomfort can end up worsening your pain and cause additional problems.

Can core exercises help?

Yes. Because no one muscle is dedicated to supporting the lower back, a program addressing a variety of core muscles is best. When done regularly, our gentle core stretches and exercises may help you avoid low back pain entirely. If you have chronic low back pain, they might also help you ease it—and put a stop to future recurrences. Before you jump in, though, be sure to read "Tailoring gentle core exercises to your abilities," page 8.

Merely making muscles strong isn't enough. One goal of our exercises is enhancing core stability—that is, your control over the position and movement of the center of your body. Recently, researchers crunching data from five randomized, controlled trials of people who had chronic lower back pain (pain lasting more than three months) compared core stability programs to general exercise programs. At follow-up points ranging from one to eight weeks, the core work proved to ease pain more effectively, and the researchers found it might improve physical function, too.

Flexibility matters, also. Tight muscles contribute to sore backs. They limit your range of motion, shortening your stride or reach, for example, and making it hard to sit or stand with good posture. Poor posture can cause backaches, too. Stretching regularly helps counter these problems.

Gentle core workouts aren't the only way to help ease your pain. Yoga and Pilates are excellent choices, too. Simpler still is walking. A 2013 trial comparing a walking program to a muscle-strengthening program for the back offered good news all around. At the end of six weeks, participants in both groups—a total of 52 sedentary people ages 18 to 65 who suffered from chronic low back pain—had improved in many ways, including the distance they could walk in six minutes, muscle endurance, and measures of function and disability. This was true no matter which program they took part in.

This section delves into why having a strong, flexible core matters in daily life and spotlights important core muscles, bones, and joints.

How a strong core benefits you

Think of your core muscles as the sturdy central link connecting your upper and lower body. The forces that propel your movements originate in your core, or transfer through it on the way to an end destination.

If you were pitching a baseball, for example, the complete arc of the movement—known as the kinetic chain—would run from the ground through your legs, hips, trunk and back, shoulder, elbow, and wrist in an even transfer of force. A hitch in the chain—a weak hip, perhaps—undercuts the strength of the movement and may start a chain of misalignments in joints and limbs that lay the groundwork for injuries over time. No matter where a motion starts, it ripples upward and downward to adjoining links of the chain. Thus, weak, tight, or inflexible core muscles can impair how well your arms and legs function. That saps power from many of the moves you make.

Conversely, properly building up your core cranks up the power as you move. Rippling abs alone won't suffice. Overtraining abdominal muscles while snubbing muscles of the back and hip can set you up for injuries and a sore back.

What's more, a strong core enhances balance and stability. Thus, it can help prevent falls that may lead to bruises and fractures. In fact, a strong, flexible, and well-balanced core underpins almost everything you do, from rising from a chair to strolling down the block or engaging in sports or any number of other activities.

▪ **Everyday acts.** Bending to put on shoes or scoop up a package, turning to look behind you, sitting in a chair, or simply standing still—these are just a few

A cure for "sitting disease"?

"Sitting disease" is a not-quite-medical phrase that captures a list of ailments worsened by sedentary habits. Prolonged sitting—an apt description of modern work and home lives for many people—harms us in many ways, according to recent research.

Extended sitting contributes to a worse ratio of good-to-bad cholesterol, slows the clearance of glucose (sugar) from the bloodstream, and reduces insulin sensitivity, all of which hike up your risks for heart disease, stroke, and type 2 diabetes. Waistlines widen, too, with implications reaching well beyond whether you can wriggle into your current wardrobe.

A 2012 study of more than 220,000 Australian adults ages 45 or older found that the risk of a premature death from all causes increased with the amount of time subjects spent seated throughout the course of the day. Mortality rose 15% among participants who sat eight to 11 hours per day, and 40% among

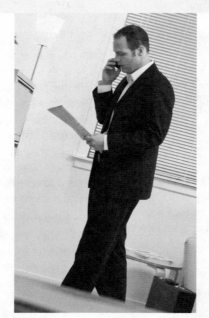

Thinkstock

people who sat 11-plus hours per day, compared with those who sat less than four hours per day.

Why does prolonged sitting have such negative health consequences? One explanation is that it relaxes your largest muscles. When muscles relax, they take up very little glucose from the blood, raising your risk of type 2 diabetes. In addition, the enzymes that break down blood fats (triglycerides) plummet, causing levels of the "good" cholesterol, HDL, to fall, too. The result? Higher risk of heart disease.

Given the research, breaking up long blocks of sitting to flex your muscles seems like a wise move for all of us. Take your phone calls standing up. Use a standing desk. Hold treadmill meetings or walking meetings. Sit on a stability ball to work or watch TV. Cut back on TV in favor of more brisk strolls or bike rides. And, yes, do core exercises.

---

of many mundane actions that rely on your core and that you might not notice until they become difficult or painful. Even basic activities of daily living—bathing or dressing, for example—call on your core.

■ **On-the-job tasks.** Jobs that involve lifting, twisting, and standing all rely on core muscles. But less strenuous tasks—like sitting at your desk for hours—engage your core as well. Phone calls, typing, computer use, and similar work can make back muscles surprisingly stiff and sore, particularly if you're not strong enough to practice good posture and aren't taking sufficient breaks.

■ **A healthy back.** Low back pain—a debilitating, sometimes excruciating problem affecting four out of five Americans at some point in their lives—may be prevented by exercises that promote well-balanced, resilient core muscles. When back pain strikes, a regimen of core exercises and walking is often prescribed to relieve it, coupled with medications, physical therapy, or other treatments.

■ **Sports and other pleasurable activities.** Golfing, tennis or other racquet sports, biking, running, swimming, baseball, volleyball, kayaking, rowing, and

many other athletic activities are powered by a strong core. Less often mentioned are sexual activities, which call for core power and flexibility, too.

■ **Housework, fix-it work, and gardening.** Bending, lifting, twisting, carrying, hammering, reaching overhead—even vacuuming, mopping, and dusting are acts that spring from, or pass through, the core.

■ **Balance and stability.** Your core stabilizes your body, enabling you to move in any direction, even on the bumpiest terrain, or stand in one spot without losing your balance. Viewed this way, core exercises can lessen your risk of falling.

■ **Good posture.** Weak core muscles contribute to slouching. Good posture trims your silhouette and projects confidence. More importantly, it lessens wear and tear on the spine and allows you to breathe deeply. Good posture helps you gain full benefits from the effort you put into exercising, too.

Major core muscles

Which muscles actually constitute your core? Reaching from your thighs to the bottom of your breastbone, your core spans muscles, bones, and joints in your abdomen, back, sides, pelvis, buttocks, and hips (see Figure 1, page 2). It doesn't stop there, though. A few muscles higher up on the back—the trapezius and latissimus dorsi—are supporting players that contribute to core stability. Here is an introduction to the major muscles that our gentle core exercises focus on.

In the abdomen

Exercise enthusiasts refer to the quartet of abdominal muscle groups simply as "abs." In fact, people do that even when singling out particular muscles like the rectus abdominis, a spotlight-hogger for its role in creating the "six-pack" or even "eight-pack" abs sported by lean, chiseled athletes and actors. The four groups are as follows:

- **rectus abdominis** (middle front)—a pair of long, vertical straps of muscle running from sternum (breastbone) and ribs to pubic bone, which enable you to flex your trunk
- **external obliques** (both sides)—two large, flat muscles that enable you to twist your torso
- **internal obliques** (both sides, underneath the external obliques)—two smaller, flat muscles that enable you to twist your torso
- **transversus abdominis** (front and back, underneath the internal obliques)—a wide, flat girdle of muscle wrapping around the torso, which stabilizes your core.

In the back

The erector spinae, a group of multiple vertical muscles collectively stretching along the entire back, help you straighten your back and stand upright with good posture.

In the pelvis, buttocks, and hips

The gluteus maximus, gluteus medius, and gluteus minimus are often referred to collectively as your "glutes" or "gluteals." The glutes and other muscles in this region, which straddles the realm from the hip joints to the muscles of the back, include these:

- **gluteus maximus** (buttocks)—two bulky muscles that permit you to powerfully extend the hip and rotate the thigh

- **gluteus medius and minimus** (buttocks)—four fan-shaped muscles, which let you rotate the hip, push your thigh away from the centerline of your body, and stabilize your pelvis while standing
- **iliopsoas** (pelvis and hips)—actually two muscle groups, the iliacus and the psoas, that reach down from the mid-spine and wrap around the hip joint to the thighbone, allowing you to rotate the pelvis, bend at the hips, and stabilize your body when you stand
- **quadratus lumborum** (pelvis and hips)—either of two straps of muscle (one on each side of the body) that

Figure 2: Regions of the spine

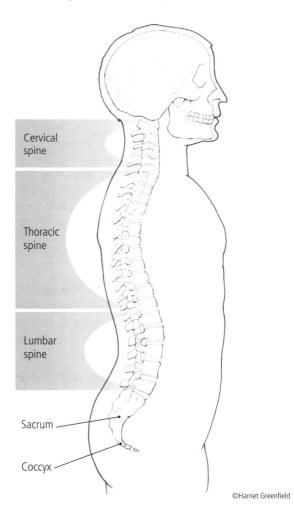

Cervical spine

Thoracic spine

Lumbar spine

Sacrum

Coccyx

©Harriet Greenfield

Core work supports the spine, especially the thoracic and the lumbar regions. Low back pain often originates in the lumbar area, which extends from the bottom of your rib cage to your sacrum (the triangular bone found between your hip bones) and includes the lowest five mobile vertebrae.

stabilize the pelvis and permit you bend to the sides and slightly backward, as well as hike up each hip.

Beyond muscles

While core muscles are essential to movement, they can't do all the work by themselves. The spine, pelvis, and hip joints, plus other structures in your body's core, are equally essential to standing, sitting, and moving.

Thirty-three interlocked vertebrae form the spine, a bony column that flexes along nearly all of its length. Vertebrae are divided into five regions. The top three regions are the cervical spine (neck), thoracic spine, and lumbar spine, the hot spot for lower back injuries and pain (see Figure 2, page 5). Sandwiched between the vertebrae in these regions are shock-absorbing discs that enable mobility. The bottom two regions form the sacrum, a triangular bone that connects to the pelvic girdle, and the short tail of the coccyx. Both consist of fused vertebrae and no discs, so this part of the spine is not flexible.

The bony girdle of the pelvis acts as the base of your core. The hip joints—two sockets that the balls at the top of the thighbones fit into neatly—are sited in the lower third of the pelvis, toward the front.

▶ Don't ignore your pelvic floor: Exercises to prevent or treat stress incontinence

One essential set of core muscles is often ignored even by exercise mavens. This sling of muscles and ligaments, called the pelvic floor, stretches from the pubic bone to the tailbone. It helps support the bladder and other pelvic organs.

When you urinate, your body relaxes the pelvic floor muscles and the two sphincter muscles that cinch the neck of the bladder. If pregnancy, childbirth, aging, or excess weight weakens the pelvic floor muscles, one set of roadblocks that helps prevent urine leaks is compromised, and the bladder may slip downward. Often, leaks start occurring when you jump, cough, laugh, or exert yourself in ways that put pressure on your abdomen. This common problem is called stress incontinence.

Strengthening pelvic floor muscles can help relieve stress incontinence in many women. In men, strengthening these muscles and other behavioral treatments, such as delaying bathroom trips to retrain the bladder, helped cut urine leaks after prostate surgery by half.

While no studies focus on posture and pelvic prolapse, holding your body upright may matter, too, since slouching could put pressure on the pelvic floor. That's one more potential reason to strengthen core muscles and practice good posture often.

Find the right muscles

Kegel exercises can help tune up pelvic floor muscles if done regularly. First, you need to pinpoint the right muscles by following these directions.

• Empty your bladder.

• Tighten the muscles you would use to avoid passing gas. If you're a woman, it may help to imagine tightening your vagina around a tampon. (An older tip—engaging the muscles you use to stop a stream of urine—has been discredited.) Generally, you should feel like you are pulling in the anal area.

• Now practice tightening, holding, and releasing the muscles. As you do this, try not to contract abdominal or leg muscles—or, indeed, any other muscles. It may help to put your hand on your belly so you can sense whether you're tightening your abs. If you're still not sure you have the right set of muscles, biofeedback can help you learn to do Kegels correctly. Talk to your doctor about this.

A simple pelvic floor exercise

Step 1. Pull in the pelvic floor muscles.

Step 2. Hold for a count of three.

Step 3. Release and relax for a count of three.

Step 4. Do 10 to 15 times.

Practice these exercises three times a day, preferably once while lying down, once while sitting, and once while standing.

While pelvic floor exercises may take three to six weeks to work, you may notice improvement sooner.

Need more help?

Talk to your doctor about other options if these exercises aren't enough. Reasons for urinary incontinence vary, and more than one problem may be involved. A thorough exam will help determine causes and identify the right treatment. Often, a doctor can suggest healthy habits and behavioral changes to help curb urine leaks, possibly in combination with medications, surgery, or other strategies.

Beyond the core: Why exercise?

Regular exercise will help you feel, think, and look better. Strong evidence from thousands of studies shows that engaging in regular exercise, including but not limited to core work, offers a host of health benefits. Among other things, it

- lowers your risks for early death, heart disease, stroke, type 2 diabetes, high blood pressure, high cholesterol, colon and breast cancers, and metabolic syndrome (a complex problem that increases the risk for stroke, heart disease, and diabetes by blending three or more of the following factors: high blood pressure, high triglycerides, low HDL cholesterol, a large waistline, and difficulty regulating blood sugar)
- strengthens muscles, lungs, and heart
- eases depression and improves mood
- helps prevent falls that can lead to debilitating fractures and loss of independence
- helps keep you from gaining weight or regaining pounds you've lost
- takes a load off aching hips and knees by strengthening supporting muscles
- boosts mental sharpness in older adults

- enables some people to cut back on medications they take, thereby easing unwanted side effects and saving money.

Moderate evidence suggests that regular exercise also

- improves functional abilities in older adults—that is, being able to walk up stairs or through a store as you do your shopping, heft groceries, rise from a chair without help, and perform a multitude of other activities that permit independence or bring joy to our lives
- helps lessen abdominal obesity, which plays a role in many serious ailments, including heart disease, diabetes, and stroke
- maintains or boosts bone density (provided the exercises are weight-bearing, meaning they work against gravity)
- lowers risk for hip fractures
- leads to better sleep
- lowers risk for endometrial cancer.

The Physical Activity Guidelines for Americans from the U.S. Department of Health and Human Services recommend 150 minutes of moderate intensity activity a week or 75 minutes of vigorous exercise (or an equivalent mix of the two).

Inside each hip joint, tough, flexible tissue called cartilage cushions the junction between bones and absorbs synovial fluid, a lubricant that helps protect against the wear and tear of friction. Ligaments made of strong, usually inelastic, tissue bind and stabilize the joint. In addition, throughout your core, flexible cords of tissue called tendons tether muscle to bone. Your brain coordinates lightning-quick signals passing along nerve pathways that instruct opposing muscles to contract and relax. The muscles tug on tendons attached to bones, allowing you to walk and jump, dance and run, twist and bend. ▼

Tailoring gentle core exercises to your abilities

While it's tempting to skip right to the workouts, it's best to think about safety first. In this section you'll find information on when you should talk to your doctor before beginning a new routine. You'll also find a list of warning signs that should prompt a call to a doctor (see "Warning signs," page 11) and tips on adapting the workouts to your needs and abilities.

Should you check with your doctor first?

Almost anyone can safely and comfortably do the simple exercises we've selected for our gentle core workouts. But you might find certain exercises especially challenging if you are very out of shape because of illness, a recent hospitalization, or just way too much couch-potato time. Similarly, if arthritis or inactivity has left your muscles and joints especially stiff, you may find it hard to do certain exercises or stretches. Depending on health issues, you may need to check with a doctor to see if you need to modify any of the gentle core exercises or avoid them altogether.

If you are healthy and normally active, odds are good you can undertake the gentle core exercises we've chosen without difficulty, particularly if you start with the Office Workout (page 19) or the Level 1 exercises in the Home Workout (page 24) and work up gradually to the more challenging Level 2 exercises that are also provided in the Home Workout.

If you're in doubt, we recommend using the Physical Activity Readiness Questionnaire For Everyone (PAR-Q+), a tool developed by the Canadian Society for Exercise Physiology, to help you determine whether you should talk to your doctor before embarking on, or ramping up, any exercise program, including our program of gentle core exercises. You can find it at www.health.harvard.edu/PAR-Q.

Whether or not you use the PAR-Q+, we recommend talking to a doctor about whether you should observe any limitations if any of the following apply:

- You've had hip surgery.
- You've been experiencing pain in your hip joints or back.
- You have a chronic or unstable health condition, such as heart disease, or you have several risk factors for heart disease, a respiratory ailment, high blood pressure, osteoporosis, or diabetes.

If you do need to speak to a doctor, we suggest that you bring or fax the core workout pages and ask if you can safely follow the program described. Your doctor may feel that the exercises are fine, or may modify certain exercises to make them safer for you. If necessary, your doctor can refer you to a physiatrist, a physical therapist, or another health care specialist for further evaluation. Occasionally, a doctor may recommend working out with the supervision of an experienced personal trainer or health professional (see "Exercise professionals," page 9).

How to adapt the routines

Assuming you've got the green light from your doctor to start exercising, monitor yourself as you go along to make sure you don't run into trouble. Use the strategies below if you encounter difficulties with the exercises or stretches. If you have very significant limitations from illness or disability, consider working with a physical therapist or personal trainer to further modify this gentle core program.

Does a medical condition cause you pain?

- Take a warm shower or bath before doing gentle core exercises or stretches to make your muscles more pliable.
- Make sure your mat is well-padded if you are doing floor work.
- If your pain results from arthritis, try the two-hour pain rule recommended by the Arthritis Founda-

Exercise professionals

In case you need extra help adapting the program, here is a brief explanation of the skills offered by, and training required of, various health and exercise professionals.

Physiatrists, also known as rehabilitation physicians, are board-certified medical doctors who specialize in treating nerve, muscle, and bone conditions that affect movement. Back problems, knee or shoulder injuries, debilitating arthritis or obesity, and stroke are a few examples. A physiatrist can tailor an exercise prescription to enhance recovery after surgery or an injury, or to help you work out despite pain or limited movement. He or she can also tell you whether certain types of exercise will be helpful or harmful given your specific health history.

Physical therapists help restore abilities to people with health conditions or injuries affecting muscles, joints, bones, or nerves. Their expertise can be valuable if, for instance, you have suffered a lingering sprain or are recovering from a heart attack or hip replacement. Some specialize in cardio-pulmonary rehabilitation, orthopedics, sports medicine, geriatrics, or other areas. After receiving a bachelor's degree, physical therapists must graduate from an accredited physical therapy program. Most accredited programs in the United States offer doctoral degrees. Additionally, physical therapists must pass a national exam given by the Federation of State Boards of Physical Therapy and be licensed by their state. Specialists complete advanced training and additional national exams to become board-certified.

Physical therapy assistants provide physical therapy services under the supervision of a physical therapist. They must complete a two-year associate's degree, pass a national exam, and, in most states, be licensed.

Clinical exercise physiologists work with people who have chronic diseases, such as cardiovascular disease, lung ailments, and metabolic disorders. They work in a medically supervised environment under the direction of a licensed physician. To qualify, they must hold a master's degree in exercise physiology, movement science, or kinesiology, and either be licensed under state law or hold a national certification, such as the ACSM's Certified Clinical Exercise Specialist or Registered Clinical Exercise Physiologist.

Personal trainers are fitness specialists who can help ensure that you're doing exercises properly. While encouraging and motivating you, they can fine-tune your form, especially helpful in core work because subtle movements can make an exercise effective or ineffective. Personal trainers teach new skills, change up routines to beat boredom, and safely push you to the next level.

No national licensing requirements exist for personal trainers, although standards for the accrediting fitness organizations that train them have been set by the National Commission for Certifying Agencies. Two well-respected organizations that offer certification and programs of study for personal trainers are the American College of Sports Medicine (ACSM) and the American Council on Exercise (ACE); others include the National Council on Strength and Fitness (NCSF), the National Strength and Conditioning Association (NSCA), and the National Academy of Sports Medicine (NASM). All fitness organizations have different requirements for training and expertise. Some trainers specialize in working with particular populations—for example, athletes or older adults—and may have taken courses and possibly certifying exams in those areas.

tion. Accept that some short-lived discomfort is likely when you exercise, especially if you haven't been active. However, if you feel more pain two hours after you finish exercising than before starting, you probably overdid it. Pare back to the point where this is no longer true (for example, by doing fewer reps or a less challenging exercise). Step up your level of exercise very gradually, keeping the two-hour rule in mind. Remember: staying active lessens arthritis (as well as low back pain) in the long run, while protecting independence and keeping you healthier over all.

• Work with your doctor to better control pain. Be aware of any dizziness or drowsiness from medications that might lead to falls, though, and report it

to your doctor. Choosing the right type and level of pain relief may require tinkering.

• Seek ways to reduce pain that do not involve medication. Acupuncture shows promise in easing chronic low back pain and osteoarthritis of the knee. Gentle self-massage and applications of cold or heat may help, though this depends on the underlying problem causing your pain. Explore these and other options with your doctor to be sure they fit your situation.

Are you finding it hard to do gentle core exercises?

• Start with the easier exercises. All exercises in the Office Workout are simple, as are all the stretches in both the Office Stretch and Home Stretch. In the

Home Workout, begin with the Level 1 exercises, mastering them before you move on to Level 2.

• Choose just two core exercises to fit into each day instead of aiming for an entire workout. For the simplest exercises, see the Office Workout and "Easiest abdominal exercises" (page 18).

Are you feeling very stiff?

• For the first two weeks, until your body begins to feel more limber, focus only on gentle core stretches (see the Office Stretch, page 22, and the Home Stretch, page 36). Then you can start folding in easy gentle core exercises from the Office Workout and "Easiest abdominal exercises" (page 18).

• Try doing your stretches after you have a warm shower or bath to loosen up your muscles.

Are you struggling to do all the repetitions (reps) that make up one set?

• When an exercise feels especially hard, perform fewer reps, stopping when you can no longer maintain good form. (For definitions of terms like "reps" and "sets," see "What does the terminology in the instructions mean?" on page 13.) Build strength by adding one more rep of the exercise during each session of core work—or every other session if you need more time to build up—until you can do the full number of reps comfortably. Only then should you add another set, if called for in the instructions.

Are you having trouble holding a position for the full number of seconds recommended?

• If even one plank knocks you out, dial down the number of seconds you hold it: aim for 10 seconds one week, then try to bump up to 15 seconds the following week. Use the same rule for stretches. Again, good form always beats length of seconds held.

Do you need to modify a movement or position?

• While good form requires closely adhering to exercise instructions, you should take a movement only as far as is comfortable for you. For example, when doing the standing knee lift (page 19), lift your knee only six inches if that's all you can manage at first.

• Sometimes small adjustments help. For example, the

front plank on desk (page 21) will be easier if the surface you lean on is high; it's more challenging if you're leaning on a lower table, desk, or countertop.

• Take stretches only to the point of mild tension, never pain. The child's pose and cobbler's pose stretches can be made easier with a rolled towel or pillows, as explained in the instructions for these stretches.

Are your muscles sore after exercise?

• Whenever you start doing a new set of exercises, you may feel a bit sore the next day or two. Delayed-onset muscle soreness is a normal response to taxing muscles. Usually, it peaks 24 to 48 hours after a workout before gradually easing, then disappearing entirely in another day or so. By contrast, sudden, sharp, or long-lasting pain should prompt you to call a doctor for advice (see "Warning signs," page 11).

• If your muscles feel really sore a day or two after a core workout, you probably overdid it. Dial down your core work next time by using Level 1 exercises, performing fewer reps, or holding a position for fewer seconds.

10 tips for doing gentle core work safely and effectively

To get the best results from our gentle core exercises and stretches, follow these 10 tips:

1. **Form first.** Good form means aligning your body as described in the exercise instructions and moving smoothly through an exercise. Read the "Tips and techniques" section of each exercise carefully for helpful cues on correct alignment. Also see "Posture and alignment" (page 16).

2. **Reps (or time held) second.** Quality trumps quantity. Do only as many repetitions (reps) as you can manage with excellent form. Likewise, hold a position only for as long as you can manage with excellent form. Plan to work up to the full number of reps or seconds gradually.

3. **Feel no pain.** Core work shouldn't hurt. Stop if you feel pain (especially lower back pain). Check your form and try again. If pain persists, check with a doctor or physical therapist before repeating that exercise.

▶ Warning signs

Call a doctor for advice if you experience any of these warning signs during or after exercise:

✔ sudden, sharp, or intense pain

✔ pain lasting one or two weeks (as distinct from delayed-onset muscle soreness, a response to working your muscles that usually peaks 24 to 48 hours after a workout, then gradually abates)

✔ dizziness; faintness; chest pain, pressure, heaviness, or tightness; or significant or persistent shortness of breath

✔ in hot, humid weather, signs of overheating such as headache, dizziness, nausea, faintness, cramps, or palpitations.

4. **Photos tell only part of the story.** Photos can make core work look easier than it actually is. Carefully read instructions in the "Tips and techniques" section of each exercise, and check out "The right (and wrong) way to do two gentle core moves," page 16.

5. **Brace yourself.** Tighten your core muscles before starting the "Movement" in each exercise. Here's how: while sitting, standing, or lying on your back, gently but firmly tighten your abdominal muscles, drawing your navel in toward the small of your back. Tuck in your tailbone slightly, too. Once you're braced, a gentle push from any direction should not cause you to lose your balance. Some trainers suggest imagining that you're pulling in your muscles to zip up a tight pair of jeans. Either way, practice makes perfect. Try bracing or zipping up for 10 seconds at a time while breathing normally.

6. **If it's too easy, move up.** As it feels easier to do exercises with good form, first add reps to complete a full set, or add seconds if the exercise calls for you to hold a position. Next, you can add sets (up to two, if called for in the instructions). Then move on to Level 2 exercises, if that's an option. As you move up to more challenging exercises, leave the simpler ones behind to make the most efficient use of your exercise time.

7. **Be balanced.** When possible, do a pair of exercises with opposing movements, such as standing hamstring curl (page 20) and standing knee lift (page 19), or ball squeeze (page 30) and standing side leg lift (page 19). This helps create balance in muscle groups. It aids in injury prevention and is often used in rehabilitation. As you'll find, the exercises in the Office Workout and Home Workout strengthen the front, back, inner, and outer leg muscles, as well as working hip, buttock, abdominal, and back muscles. Looking for single exercises that work several muscle groups at once? Try front planks (page 34), side planks (page 31), and the opposite arm and leg raise (page 26).

8. **Be flexible.** Core flexibility is as important as core strength. In fact, too much strength without flexibility can make your back throb and interfere with smooth, powerful moves in sports like tennis and golf. So don't skimp on stretches when you're shoehorning core work into your day. Do a full Office Stretch or Home Stretch at least twice a week.

9. **Warm muscles before stretching.** Muscles are a bit like taffy—you'll get a better stretch if your body is warmed up. You'll be less likely to injure yourself, too. If you stretch after doing core exercises or at least five minutes of walking or another activity, you're all set. If you're only doing stretches, march in place for several minutes while swinging your arms or dance to a few songs to warm up muscles.

10. **Practice often.** You'll notice real gains if you practice core exercises three or more times a week. One helpful strategy is to sprinkle core work throughout the day—for example, a set of clams (page 32) plus a front plank on knees (page 34) before dressing, a set of chair stands (page 21) after lunch, an Office Workout or Office Stretch during a short break, or a calming Home Stretch before bed. ◗

Structuring your workout: Four commonly asked questions

Before you begin the exercises, you may have questions about how to fit core work into your overall exercise routine, what equipment you need, and how to interpret the directions in the exercises themselves.

1. How should core work fit into your overall exercise plans?

Fitting core work into a broader exercise plan will give you the biggest bang for your buck in terms of health benefits (see "Beyond the core: Why exercise?" on page 7). A well-rounded exercise plan has several facets, according to the Physical Activity Guidelines for Americans from the U.S. Department of Health and Human Services, which recommends the following:

- Accumulate at least two-and-a-half hours (150 minutes) of moderate aerobic activity per week, or one-and-a-quarter hours (75 minutes) of vigorous activity per week, or an equivalent combination of the two. During moderate activity, such as a brisk walk, you can talk, but not sing; during vigorous activity, such as running, you can't say more than a few words without catching your breath (see Table 1, at left). Walking, running, biking, swimming, cross-country skiing, tennis, rowing, and many additional activities offer aerobic benefits.
- Do strength-training sessions twice a week for all major muscle groups, including your core.
- Add balance exercises if you're an older adult at risk for falling.

Core work falls under the second and third categories: strength training and enhancing balance. Many of the exercises we've selected tone more than just core muscles: for example, chair stands strengthen muscles throughout your legs, while planks work some arm and back muscles as well as abdominal muscles. However, gentle core exercises cannot fulfill all your strength-training needs. To meet the recommendations, you'll need to add some strength-training exercises to ensure that you're working all major muscle groups twice a week (see "Resources," page 44).

When deciding how to fit core work into your weekly activities, consider which of the following options best fits your schedule and goals. Core work doesn't have to take a lot of time. Slipping in exercises and stretches during the day or adding a few core exercises to your usual routine requires just a few minutes.

■ **Do a short workout.** The three groups of exercises on page 18 can each be treated as a short workout. Estimate 10 minutes for one set.

■ **Perform a complete workout.** Aim to do a core workout two to three times a week. Start with Level 1

Table 1: How hard are you working?

INTENSITY	IT FEELS...	YOU ARE...
Light	Easy	• Breathing easily • Warming up, but not yet sweating • Able to talk—or even sing an aria, if you have the talent
Light to moderate	You're working, but not too hard	• Breathing easily • Sweating lightly • Still finding it easy to talk or sing
Moderate	You're working	• Breathing faster • Starting to sweat more • Able to talk, not able to sing
Moderate to high	You're really working	• Huffing and puffing • Sweating • Able to talk in short sentences, but concentrating more on exercise than conversation
High	You're working very hard, almost out of steam	• Breathing hard • Sweating hard • Finding talking difficult

exercises, taking as long as you need to work up to the recommended number of reps and sets. When this becomes easy, substitute Level 2 exercises. Changing workouts can help keep you motivated.

■ **Sprinkle in core work.** Add short bursts of core work throughout the day by choosing exercises or stretches to do a few times a day. You can do this daily, or start slowly by writing a reminder on your calendar—say, every Monday and Thursday—then gradually folding core exercise into additional days.

■ **Tack core work on to strength sessions.** When you do your twice-weekly strength-training sessions—assuming you're following exercise recommendations!—add two extra core exercises to your regimen. This option is an excellent fallback position during especially busy weeks. During less busy weeks, try to step it up again by doing a core workout or sprinkling bursts of core work throughout your day.

2. What equipment will you need?

Almost all of our gentle core exercises rely on body weight and gravity alone. Practically no equipment is needed, with these exceptions:

■ **Ball.** For the ball squeeze exercise (page 30), you'll need a rubber or plastic ball about the size of a child's soccer ball. Many supermarkets and big box stores carry these inexpensive balls in a toy section.

■ **Chair.** Many of our exercises call for a sturdy chair that won't tip over easily. A plain wooden dining chair without arms or heavy padding works well. Do not use a desk chair with wheels! In most cases, you can put your hands on a countertop or desk to help you balance if a chair isn't available.

■ **Mat.** Choose a nonslip, well-padded mat for floor exercises and stretches. Yoga mats are readily available, though these mats tend to be thin. A thick carpet or towels will do in a pinch.

■ **Yoga strap (optional).** A yoga strap—a cotton or nylon strap of six feet or longer—can be used to help you position your body properly during certain stretches, such as the hamstring stretch lying down. Choose a strap with a D-ring or buckle fastener on one end. This allows you to put a loop around a foot or leg and then grasp the other end of the strap.

▶ **Why not just do a few sit-ups?**

Once, sit-ups ruled in dusty school gyms, and planks were merely flooring. Now exercises known as planks have claimed the spotlight as core workout stars, while old standards such as sit-ups and crunches have fallen out of favor. Why the shift?

First, sit-ups may injure your back by pushing your curved spine against the floor, and also by overworking the hip flexor muscles, which run from the thighs to the lumbar spine of the lower back. When these muscles are too strong or overly tight, they tug on lumbar vertebrae, which can be a source of lower back discomfort.

Second, planks recruit a better balance of muscles on the front, sides, and back of the body than sit-ups, which target just a few muscles. Remember, your core goes far beyond the abs of six-pack fame.

Third, physical activities call on your muscles to work together, not in isolation. Sit-ups or crunches cherry-pick a few muscle groups to strengthen. Our core workouts, including planks, stress dynamic patterns of movement used in many activities that build up your entire core.

3. What does the terminology in the instructions mean?

Every gentle core exercise and stretch includes certain instructions, which are explained below.

■ **Repetitions (reps).** Each rep is a single, complete movement for one exercise. If you cannot do all the reps at first, just do as many as you can manage with good form. Gradually increase reps as you improve.

■ **Set.** One set is a specific number of repetitions. In our gentle core exercises, a set is usually eight to 10 reps (the exception is a few very challenging exercises, such as planks, which call for one rep). Generally, we suggest doing one to two sets. Just as with reps, only do the number of sets you can manage with good form and work your way up over time.

■ **Hold.** Hold tells you the number of seconds to pause while holding a pose during an exercise. You'll see this in stretches, which are held for 10 to 30 seconds, and in plank exercises, for example. Start with a comfortable number of seconds, then work up. Holding for the full recommended time will give you the best results from the stretch or exercise.

■ **Rest.** A rest is recommended between sets of certain exercises to give your muscles a chance to recharge, which helps you maintain good form. We specify a range of time to rest between sets. How much of this time you need will differ depending on your level of fitness and how challenging the exercise is. No rest is needed during warm-ups and stretches, or when you are not doing a second set of exercises.

■ **Tempo.** This provides a count for the key movements in an exercise. For example, the 2-2 tempo in the standing side leg lift (page 19) requires you to count to two as you lift your leg straight out to the side, then count to two as you lower your leg to the floor. The 2-4-2 tempo in the bridge (page 29) requires you to count to two while lifting your hips off the floor, hold for a count of four, then count to two while lowering your hips to the floor. At first, it helps to count while watching or listening to the seconds tick by on a clock to avoid hurrying. If you can no longer maintain the recommended tempo, your muscles are fatigued. Stop that particular exercise even if you haven't finished all of the reps.

■ **Starting position.** This describes how to position your body before starting the movement of the exercise.

■ **Movement.** This explains how to perform one complete repetition correctly.

■ **Tips and techniques.** We offer two or three pointers to help you maintain good form and reap the greatest gains from the exercise.

4. How can you measure gains?

Time can pass awfully slowly when you're hoping to see results after embarking on a new exercise regimen. But if you do gentle core work consistently, you can start to see progress in as little as two to four weeks; if you start more slowly or exercise less consistently, progress will take longer. Best results are obtained when you do workouts or exercises several times a week and step up to more challenging exercises when you've mastered the easier ones.

To monitor your progress, we suggest doing a baseline test of endurance, strength, flexibility, and balance before you start gentle core exercises. Only do as many reps or hold for as many seconds as you can manage with good form while following the tempo specified. If these exercises are too easy for you, step up to the Level 2 variations (see "Home Workout levels at a glance," page 24). Jot down the answers in the space provided. Then measure again every two to four weeks.

Of course, you can measure gains more informally, too, in any number of ways. Are you closer to success in the goal you set? Does your back hurt less? What tasks are you finding easier to perform? How much easier is it to bend and tie a shoelace or pick something up?

Endurance
Perform a front plank on desk (page 21), holding it for as long as you can.

Date of baseline: _____   How many seconds _____
   Date of test 1: _____   How many seconds _____
   Date of test 2: _____   How many seconds _____
   Date of test 3: _____   How many seconds _____
   Date of test 4: _____   How many seconds _____

Strength
Perform the chair stand (page 21), doing as many reps as you can.

Date of baseline: _____   How many reps _____
   Date of test 1: _____   How many reps _____
   Date of test 2: _____   How many reps _____
   Date of test 3: _____   How many reps _____
   Date of test 4: _____   How many reps _____

Flexibility
The YMCA sit-and-reach test described below is a good way to measure gains in flexibility. Ask your doctor whether you should do this test if you have low back pain. If it's okay for you to proceed, warm up for at least five minutes (walk in place, dance to a few songs) and then do either Home Stretch or Office Stretch. When you're done, perform the sit-and-reach test three times, noting the best measurement.

It helps to have a friend check measurements and make sure your legs stay straight as you reach, though without interfering with your movement. Note: If you don't have measuring tape or a yardstick, simply notice how far the tips of your fingers extend beyond a body landmark like your knees, ankles, or toes.

Challenging yourself and maintaining gains

Are you wondering when and how to progress? Or do you feel you've gone far enough and just want to maintain gains you've made? Either way, our tips below will help.

When to progress

Repeatedly challenging muscles makes them stronger. As you get stronger, exercises in your routine will become easier to do. You're ready to progress if you can manage all four of these tasks throughout each exercise:

• maintain good form

• stick to the specified tempo

• use a full, or comfortable, range of motion

• complete the suggested number of reps or hold the position for the suggested number of seconds.

How to progress

You can continue to challenge your muscles by making one of these choices:

• adding sets (up to two, if specified in the instructions)

• trying the Level 2 variation of the exercise

• moving up to a more challenging core regimen, such as the six workouts provided in the *Core Exercises* Special Health Report (see "Resources," page 44).

How to maintain gains

At some point, you may be satisfied with the gains you've made. To maintain gains, continue your routine, sticking to the highest level of challenge you've achieved.

If you get sick or take time off for other reasons, you may need to drop down a level or do fewer reps and sets before building up again.

What if you begin to feel bored? Go over your goals again. Then vary your core work by trying a new workout or selecting new exercises to do throughout the day. For options, see "Home Workout levels at a glance," page 24, and the workouts themselves, pages 19–21 and 24-35.

■ **Starting position.** First, fasten a measuring tape or yardstick to the floor by running a strip of colored tape across the 15-inch mark. Take off your shoes and sit on the floor with your legs about 12 inches apart. The yardstick should be between your legs, with the zero mark pointing toward your crotch and your heels at the 14-inch mark because they tend to slide forward a bit as you stretch.

■ **Movement.** Put one hand on top of the other, middle fingers touching. Exhale as you slowly stretch forward with arms extended and your fingertips sliding lightly along the measuring tape, yardstick, or floor. Don't bounce or jerk. Return to the starting position. Rest a few seconds and repeat. Do three sit-and-reach stretches, noting the farthest measurement.

Date of baseline: _____ How far did you stretch? _____

   Date of test 1: _____ How far did you stretch? _____

   Date of test 2: _____ How far did you stretch? _____

   Date of test 3: _____ How far did you stretch? _____

   Date of test 4: _____ How far did you stretch? _____

Balance

Core work should help improve your balance. One of the best tests for measuring gains is the single leg stance. Here's how to do it: Stand comfortably near the wall, with your arms in any position you choose. Lift one foot an inch or two off the floor so that you are balancing on the other foot. Time how long you can do this before having to put the raised foot down or touch the wall for support.

   If you can't stand on one leg, lightly touch the wall or hold the back of a chair with one or both hands for support. Use less support as you improve your balance.

Date of baseline: _____ How many seconds:

   Left foot _____ Right foot _____

Date of test 1: _____ How many seconds:

   Left foot _____ Right foot _____

Date of test 2: _____ How many seconds:

   Left foot _____ Right foot _____

Date of test 3: _____ How many seconds:

   Left foot _____ Right foot _____

Date of test 4: _____ How many seconds:

   Left foot _____ Right foot _____

   If you can hold a single leg stance for 60 seconds or more, you have excellent balance. If you can't hold it for more than 10 seconds, you are at risk for a fall. In this case, talk to your doctor about ways to improve your balance and reduce your chances of falling. ♥

Posture and alignment

Posture counts a lot when you're exercising. Aligning your body properly is the key to good form, which nets you greater gains and fewer injuries. In fact, good posture helps anytime you're moving. If one foot is always turned slightly inward, for example, it impedes power whether you're walking, going upstairs, jogging, or playing sports. Worse, it paves the way for injuries to the ankle, knee, hip, and beyond, since the effects of this physical quirk can zigzag their way up your body. Similarly, sitting up straight and comfortably aligned in a chair can make desk work feel less tiresome. Hours of computer and desk work tend to make your shoulders hunch and your head and neck jut forward uncomfortably.

Committing to core work will do much to improve your posture whether you're sitting, standing, or moving. A well-rounded set of core exercises, such as those selected for our workouts, is best. If you only pour your efforts into strengthening the most obvious set of core muscles—your abs—your back muscles will grow weaker by comparison. Then, instead of standing up straight, your body will curve forward. Likewise, your posture is thrown off kilter when muscles lose flexibility. As muscles become less flexible, they tighten and eventually shorten so that your range of motion becomes increasingly limited. Among other problems, this can cause lower back pain. That's why core stretches are so important.

The right (and wrong) way to do two gentle core moves

Good form is crucial to protecting yourself from injury and getting the most benefit from an exercise. The plank is a classic core exercise that is often done the wrong way. Even in this gentle core version (at right), it's important to maintain good form, with your body aligned, or else your core won't benefit. In the side leg lift (below), try to avoid rotating the hip and foot, or else you will throw the rest of your body out of alignment.

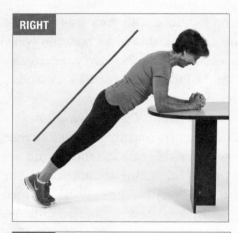

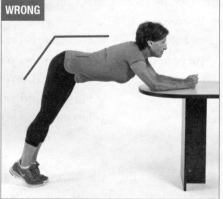

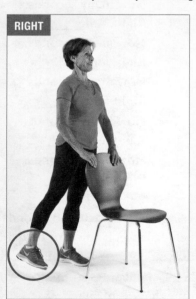

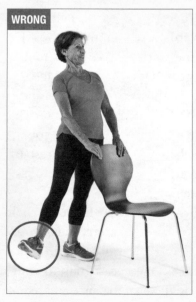

Our exercises build strength and flexibility in all your major core muscles. Doing our gentle workouts, or sprinkling several core exercises and stretches throughout your day, can help you avoid such problems.

Posture checks

Quick posture checks before and during exercise help you avoid injury and squeeze the most benefit from your workout. If possible, look in a mirror when exercising until you get the hang of it. Try to take a few moments each day to practice better posture, too.

When exercise instructions in our workouts ask you to *stand up straight*, that means
- chin parallel to the floor
- shoulders even (roll them up, back, and down to help achieve this)
- arms at your sides, elbows relaxed and even with each other
- abdominal muscles pulled in
- hips even
- knees even and pointing straight ahead
- feet pointing straight ahead
- body weight evenly distributed on both feet.

Alignment: Stay neutral

Neutral alignment is also important while exercising because it places the least amount of stress on the body. A *neutral wrist* is firm and straight, not bent upward or downward. A *neutral spine* is straight, except for the gentle, natural curves of the spine—it's not flexed or arched to overemphasize the curves of the upper or lower back.

One way to find the neutral position for your spine is to tip your pelvis forward as far as is comfortable, then tip it backward as far as is comfortable. The spot approximately in the middle should be neutral. If you're not used to standing or sitting up straight, it may take a while for this to feel natural. (When you do this, the upper back usually comes into alignment, too. But to be sure, check that your ribs are lined up with your hips, and your shoulders are even.) Maintaining a neutral spine is important, because it puts the least amount of stress on the internal organs and allows the lungs to expand fully, so your body functions better.

Neutral alignment of the body means keeping your entire body in a straight line from head to toe, except for the natural curves of the spine. ◗

Choosing which gentle core exercises to do

You can do core work anywhere—well, almost anywhere, as you'll see in our two gentle core exercise routines.

Two workouts and sets of stretches

Our first workout is called the Office Workout, because it's a short group of six simple exercises that you can easily perform at work without drawing undue attention. The exercises in the Office Workout are our simplest all-around exercises and provide an excellent way to ease into gentle core work. But just because we've designated these exercises as ways to build some movement into your work day, that doesn't mean you can't do them at home, too. Instead of doing the front plank (page 21) while leaning on your desk, for example, use the kitchen counter to support your weight while performing this exercise.

Because you should always stretch after exercising, we follow the Office Workout with the Office Stretch— a group of five simple stretches that will help counter stiffness from too many hours spent sitting.

Our second gentle core routine is called the Home Workout. Again, though we put the word "home" in the title, you don't have to limit yourself to doing it at home. These exercises are appropriate for the gym as well. To conclude, we offer you, appropriately, the Home Stretch—six stretches to help you stay flexible through your core.

Two levels of difficulty

While all of our gentle core exercises are relatively easy, we also want you to be able to move on to greater challenges as you become stronger. That's why our Home Workout includes exercises with two levels of difficulty—an easier version (Level 1) and a harder version (Level 2). The Level 2 exercises work the same muscles as the corresponding Level 1 exercises, but they pose a slightly greater challenge. You can move through them in the order we suggest or mix and match to build your own routine. Here are some suggestions. (Also see "Be balanced," page 11.)

Easiest abdominal exercises

This trio represents the simplest, easiest gentle core exercises you'll find anywhere to work your abs. This is a good way to start tuning up your core if you're very out of shape. The movements are subtle, so read carefully before you start, paying attention to our tips. **Equipment needed:** Exercise mat.
- pelvic tilt (page 27)
- alternating knee lift lying down (page 27)
- abdominal contraction (page 26).

4 excellent exercises for life: Level 1

Small package, great big bang: these four exercise stars will help you build core strength for life. **Equipment needed:** Desk (a table or countertop is fine), exercise mat, sturdy chair.
- front plank on desk (page 21)
- bridge (page 29)
- chair stand (page 21)
- abdominal contraction (page 26).

4 excellent exercises for life: Level 2

Minimal time, maximal gain: these Level 2 all-stars help you build a strong, sturdy core for life in practically no time at all. If any of these exercises are too challenging, step down to their Level 1 counterparts (see "Home Workout levels at a glance," page 24). **Equipment needed:** Exercise mat, sturdy chair.
- front plank (page 34)
- bridge with knee to chest (page 29)
- staggered chair stand (page 25)
- opposite arm and leg raise (page 26). ♥

Office Workout

Here are six exercises you can do at your desk while dressed to impress, or at home in a T-shirt and shorts. Consider this sextet your first line of defense against the "sitting disease" (see "A cure for 'sitting disease'?" on page 4). This workout is perfect for long phone calls—unless you're on Skype!

Equipment needed: Desk (a table or countertop is fine), sturdy chair that won't tilt or roll away.

---

1 Standing knee lift

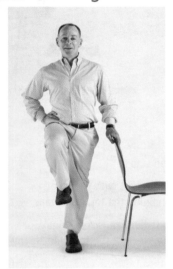

Reps: 8–10
Sets: 1–2
Tempo: 2-2
Rest: 30–90 seconds between sets

Starting position: Stand up straight with your feet together. Put your hands out to the sides for balance, elbows slightly bent, or hold the back of a chair with your left hand for support and put your right hand on your hip.

Movement: Exhale as you lift your right knee toward the ceiling as high as is comfortable, then lower the foot to the floor. This is one rep. Finish all reps, then repeat with the left leg. This completes one set.

Tips and techniques:
• Keep your chest lifted and your shoulders down and back.
• Tighten your abdominal muscles throughout.
• Tighten the buttock of your standing leg for stability.

---

2 Standing side leg lift

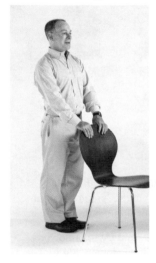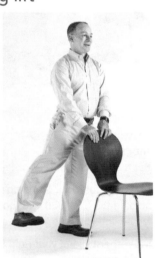

Reps: 8–10
Sets: 1–2
Tempo: 2-2
Rest: 30–90 seconds between sets

Starting position: Stand up straight behind a chair, holding the back of it with both hands. Put your feet together and evenly distribute your weight on both feet.

Movement: Slowly lift your right leg straight out to the side until your foot is about six inches off the floor. Return to the starting position. This is one rep. Finish all reps, then repeat with the left leg. This completes one set.

Tips and techniques:
• Keep your shoulders, hips, and knees aligned throughout the movement.
• Keep your spine neutral and your shoulders down and back.
• Tighten the buttock of your standing leg for stability throughout the leg lift.

3 | Standing hamstring curl

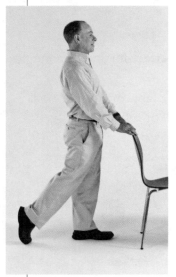 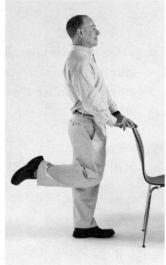

Reps: 8–10
Sets: 1–2
Tempo: 2-2
Rest: 30–90 seconds between sets

Starting position: Stand up straight behind a chair, holding the back of it with both hands. Extend your right leg behind you with your toes touching the floor.

Movement: Bend your right knee and try to bring your heel toward your right buttock. Slowly lower your foot to the floor. This is one rep. Finish all reps, then repeat with the left leg. This completes one set.

Tips and techniques:
• Maintain good posture throughout.
• Keep your hips even, tightening the buttock of the standing leg to help you balance.
• Breathe comfortably.

4 | Soccer kick

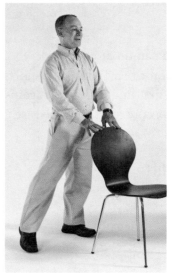 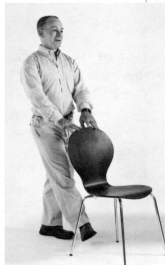

Reps: 8–10
Sets: 1–2
Tempo: 2-1-2
Rest: 30–90 seconds between sets

Starting position: Stand up straight with your feet together and your left hand holding the top of a chair.

Movement: Tighten your abdominal muscles. Point your right foot out to the right side, then lift the foot and slowly sweep it diagonally in front of you as if kicking a soccer ball with the inside of your foot. Hold. Slowly bring your foot back to the right side. This is one rep. Finish all reps, then repeat with the left leg. This completes one set.

Tips and techniques:
• Keep your hips even and maintain neutral posture throughout.
• Tighten your abdominal muscles and the buttock of the standing leg.
• Breathe comfortably.

5 Chair stand

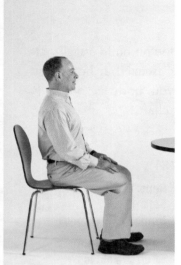 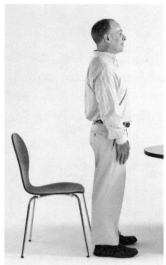

Reps: 8–10
Sets: 1
Tempo: 4-4

Starting position: Sit in a chair with your feet hip-width apart. Place your hands on your thighs.

Movement: Tighten your abdominal muscles. Exhale as you slowly stand up. Slowly sit down with control. This is one rep.

Tips and techniques:
• Press your heels against the floor and tighten your buttocks as you stand to help you balance.
• Steady yourself before you sit down.
• Exhale as you stand, inhale as you sit.

6 Front plank on desk

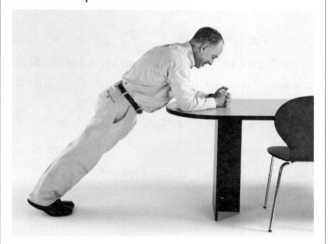

Reps: 1
Sets: 1
Hold: 15–60 seconds

Starting position: Stand facing a desk or counter with your feet together.

Movement: Tighten your abdominal muscles and lower your upper body weight onto your forearms on the desk or countertop. Clasp your hands together and align your shoulders directly over your elbows. Step back on the balls of your feet until you are balancing your body in a line like a plank. Hold. This is one rep.

Tips and techniques:
• Keep your head and spine neutral during the plank.
• Keep your shoulders down and back.
• Breathe comfortably. ♥

Office Stretch

Slip these five seated or standing stretches into your work day, or do them at home. The office stretches help ease back pain and counter stiffness that creeps up as you sit for long periods, particularly in front of a computer. Plus, they'll help you build a well-balanced, flexible core. You'll be amazed at how good stretching regularly can make your body feel.

Equipment needed: Sturdy chair.

1 Seated hamstring stretch

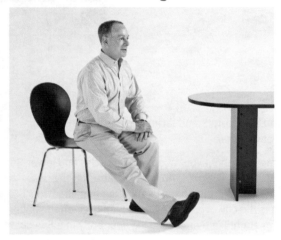

Reps: 2
Sets: 1
Hold: 10–30 seconds

Starting position: Sit up straight toward the front of a chair with your feet flat on the floor.

Movement: Extend your right leg straight in front of you with the heel grounded on the floor and toes pointing to the ceiling. Hinge forward from the hip, placing your hands on your left thigh for support. Keep your spine neutral. Hold. Repeat with the left leg. This is one rep.

Tips and techniques:
• Stretch to the point of mild tension, not pain. You should not feel any pressure behind the knee.
• Keep your shoulders down and back.
• Breathe comfortably.

2 Seated torso rotation

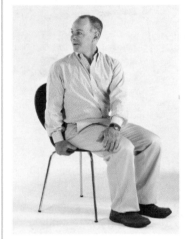

Reps: 2
Sets: 1
Hold: 10–30 seconds

Starting position: Sit up straight in a chair with your feet flat on the floor, hip-width apart, and your arms at your sides.

Movement: Slowly rotate your head and torso to the right side, placing your left hand on the outside of your right knee and your right hand next to your right hip. Hold. Slowly return to the starting position. Repeat to the left side, this time with your right hand on the outside of your left knee and your left hand next to your left hip. This is one rep.

Tips and techniques:
• Sit up straight with chest lifted, abdominal muscles braced, and shoulders down and back.
• Stretch to the point of mild tension, not pain.
• Don't hold your breath. Breathe comfortably.

3 Seated pretzel stretch

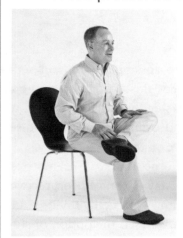

Reps: 2
Sets: 1
Hold: 10–30 seconds

Starting position: Sit up straight in a chair and rest your left ankle on your right knee. Place your hands on your thighs.

Movement: Keeping your spine neutral, slowly hinge forward from your hips until you feel mild tension in your left hip and buttock. Hold. Slowly return to the starting position. Repeat with your right ankle on your left knee. This is one rep.

Tips and techniques:

• Stretch to the point of mild tension, not pain.
• Keep your spine neutral and your shoulders down and back.
• Breathe comfortably, exhaling as you hinge forward.

4 Seated inner thigh stretch

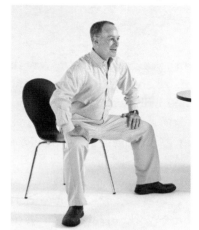

Reps: 2
Sets: 1
Hold: 10–30 seconds

Starting position: Sit up straight in a chair and open your legs as far apart as you can with knees and toes pointed out.

Movement: Put your hands on your thighs. Keeping your spine neutral, hinge forward from the hips to the point of mild tension. Hold. Return to starting position. This is one rep.

Tips and techniques:

• Stretch to the point of mild tension, not pain.
• Keep your spine neutral and your shoulders down and back.
• Breathe comfortably, exhaling as you hinge forward.

5 Standing quad stretch

Reps: 2
Sets: 1
Hold: 10–30 seconds

Starting position: Stand up straight, feet together, holding the back of a chair with both hands.

Movement: Bend your right knee and reach back with your right hand to grasp your foot, lifting it toward your right buttock. Hold. Slowly lower your foot to the floor, then switch position so that your right hand is holding the back of the chair and repeat the stretch with your left leg. This is one rep.

Tips and techniques:

• Stretch to the point of mild tension, not pain.
• If you have trouble grasping your foot, place a yoga strap around the foot to assist with the stretch.
• Breathe comfortably.

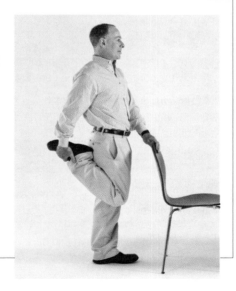

Home Workout

At home (or the gym), you have more leeway than in an office. You can lie on the carpet or on an exercise mat, and no one will give you strange looks. Here's a routine of gentle exercises to work all your core muscle groups in the abs, back, sides, pelvis, and buttocks.

Throughout, we've paired an easier Level 1 exercise with a more challenging Level 2 exercise that works the same muscles (see "Home Workout levels at a glance," below). Start with Level 1 exercises, focusing on the quality of your repetitions, rather than the quantity. Maintaining good form, posture, and alignment for fewer reps is preferable to doing a greater number of reps with poor form (see "Posture and alignment," page 16). When you master the movement and are able to do the recommended number of reps and sets fairly easily, you can move on to Level 2 exercises.

If completing the Home Workout seems overwhelming at first—as it may if you've been recovering from an illness or injury—mentally divide it into smaller chunks, and give yourself the option of stopping at the end of each one.

Equipment needed: Exercise mat, sturdy chair that won't tilt or roll away, 12-inch ball.

Home Workout levels at a glance

The following exercises come in pairs, each with an easier and harder version. **Level 1** exercises are the easier ones. **Level 2** exercises are more challenging.

LEVEL 1	PAGE	LEVEL 2	PAGE
Abdominal contraction	26	Opposite arm and leg raise	26
Ball squeeze	30	Side-lying inner thigh leg raise	30
Bridge	29	Bridge with knee to chest	29
Chair stand	25	Staggered chair stand	25
Crunch with one leg extended	28	Alternating toe taps	28
Front plank on knees	34	Front plank	34
Modified side plank	31	Side plank with bent knees	31
Pelvic tilt	27	Alternating knee lift lying down	27
Seated knee extension	33	Single leg raise	33
Side-lying leg lift	32	Clam	32

1 Level 1: Chair stand

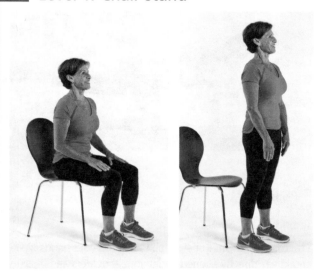

Reps: 8–10
Sets: 1
Tempo: 4-4

Starting position: Sit in a chair with your feet hip-width apart. Place your hands on your thighs.

Movement: Tighten your abdominal muscles. Exhale as you slowly stand up. Slowly sit down with control. This is one rep.

Tips and techniques:

• Press your heels against the floor and tighten your buttocks as you stand to help you balance.

• Steady yourself before you sit down.

• Exhale as you stand, inhale as you sit.

Level 2: Staggered chair stand

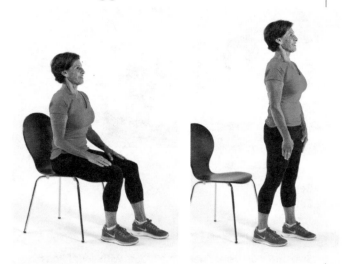

Reps: 8–10 per side
Sets: 1
Tempo: 4-4

Starting position: Sit in a chair with your feet a few inches apart and staggered so that your right heel is next to the toes of your left foot. Place your hands on your thighs.

Movement: Tighten your abdominal muscles. Exhale as you slowly stand up. Slowly sit down with control. This is one rep. Finish all reps, then repeat with your left heel next to the toes of your right foot. This completes one set.

Tips and techniques:

• Press your heels against the floor and tighten your buttocks as you stand to help you balance.

• Steady yourself before you sit down.

• Exhale as you stand, inhale as you sit.

2 | Level 1: Abdominal contraction

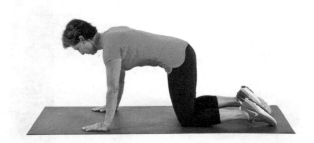

Reps: 8–10
Sets: 1–2
Tempo: 2-4-2
Rest: 30–90 seconds between sets

Starting position: Kneel on all fours with your hands and knees directly aligned under your shoulders and hips. Keep your head and spine neutral.

Movement: Exhale as you tighten your abdominal muscles by pulling them up toward your spine. Keep your spine neutral (no arching your back!). Hold. Release your abdominal muscles and return to the starting position. This is one rep.

Tips and techniques:
• This is a very subtle movement and your spine should stay still throughout the exercise.
• Breathe comfortably, exhaling as you pull your abdominal muscles in and up like a zipper.

Level 2: Opposite arm and leg raise

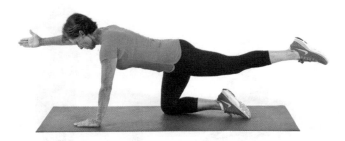

Reps: 8–10
Sets: 1
Tempo: 2-2-2

Starting position: Kneel on all fours with your hands and knees directly aligned under your shoulders and hips. Keep your head and spine neutral.

Movement: Extend your left leg off the floor behind you while reaching out in front of you with your right arm. Keeping your hips and shoulders squared, try to bring the extended leg and arm parallel to the floor. Hold. Return to the starting position, then repeat with your right leg and left arm. This is one rep.

Tips and techniques:
• Keep your shoulders and hips squared to maintain alignment throughout.
• Keep your head and spine neutral.
• Think of pulling your hand and leg in opposite directions, lengthening your torso.

3 Level 1: Pelvic tilt

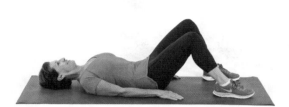

Reps: 8–10
Sets: 1–2
Tempo: 2-2-2
Rest: 30–90 seconds between sets

Starting position: Lie on your back with your knees bent, feet flat on the floor and hip-width apart. Place your arms on the floor by your sides.

Movement: Exhale as you gently tighten your abdominal muscles as if pulling your navel toward your spine, and slightly tilt your pelvis, flattening your lower back on the floor. Hold. Return to the starting position. This is one rep.

Tips and techniques:
- This is a subtle movement. Try it once with your hands on your pelvis so that you feel the pelvic tilt as you do it.
- Keep your shoulders down and back, relaxing them against the floor.
- Breathe comfortably.

Level 2: Alternating knee lift lying down

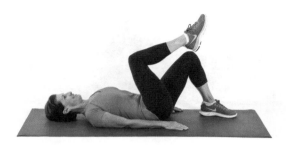

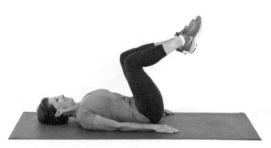

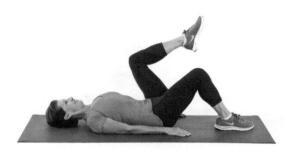

Reps: 8–10
Sets: 1–2
Tempo: 2-2-2-2
Rest: 30–90 seconds between sets

Starting position: Lie on your back with your knees bent, feet flat on the floor. Place your arms on the floor by your sides.

Movement: Tighten your abdominal muscles. Lift your right knee up toward your chest, lift your left knee up toward your chest, then lower your right foot to the floor, and lower your left foot to the floor to return to the starting position. This is one rep.

Tips and techniques:
- Keep your spine neutral throughout the four-part movement.
- Breathe comfortably, exhaling as you lift your legs and inhaling as you lower them.

4 ## Level 1: Crunch with one leg extended

Level 2: Alternating toe taps

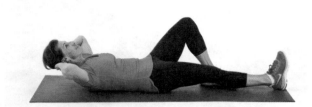

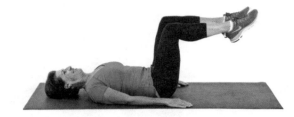

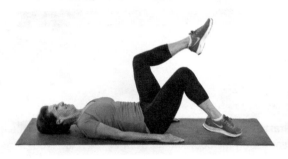

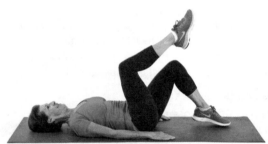

Reps: 8–10
Sets: 1
Tempo: 2-2-2

Starting position: Lie on your back with your left knee bent and foot flat on the floor. Extend your right leg. Place both hands under your head on the floor.

Movement: Exhale as you tighten your abdominal muscles and lift your head and shoulders slightly off the floor. Hold. Return to starting position. This is one rep. Finish all reps before repeating with leg positions reversed. This completes one set.

Tips and techniques:
• Breathe comfortably, exhaling as you lift your head and shoulders off the floor.
• Focus your eyes on the ceiling.
• Lift only to your comfortable range of motion.

Reps: 8–10   **Rest:** 30–90 seconds
Sets: 1–2   between sets
Tempo: 2-2

Starting position: Lie on your back, then raise your knees so that they are aligned over your hips with your legs forming a 90-degree angle at the knees. This is called a tabletop position. Your calves should be parallel to the floor. Rest your hands at your sides.

Movement: Tighten your abdominal muscles. Keeping your knees bent and your lower back flat against the floor, lower your right foot to tap the floor and then bring it back up to the starting position. Repeat with your left foot. This is one rep.

Tips and techniques:
• Keep your spine neutral—no arching your back!— throughout the movement.
• Lower each foot only as far as you comfortably can while keeping your lower back flat against the floor.
• Breathe comfortably, exhaling as you lower each foot toward the floor.

5 | Level 1: Bridge

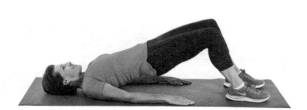

Reps: 8–10
Sets: 1–2
Tempo: 2-4-2
Rest: 30–90 seconds between sets

Starting position: Lie on your back with your knees bent and feet flat on the floor, hip-width apart. Place your arms at your sides. Relax your shoulders against the floor.

Movement: Tighten your abdominal muscles and your buttocks, then lift your hips up off the floor as high as is comfortable. Keep your hips even and spine neutral. Hold. Return to the starting position.

Tips and techniques:
• Tighten your buttocks before lifting.
• Keep your shoulders, hips, knees, and feet evenly aligned.
• Keep your shoulders down and back, relaxing them against the floor.

Level 2: Bridge with knee to chest

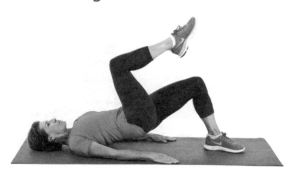

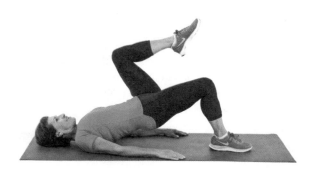

Reps: 8–10
Sets: 1
Tempo: 2-2-2-2-2-2

Starting position: Lie on your back with your knees bent and feet flat on the floor, hip-width apart. Place your arms at your sides. Relax your shoulders against the floor.

Movement: Tighten your abdominal muscles and your buttocks, then lift your hips up off the floor as high as is comfortable. Keeping your hips even and spine neutral, pull in your right knee toward your chest as far as is comfortable. Return your right foot to the floor. Pull in your left knee toward your chest as far as is comfortable. Return your left foot to the floor. Lower your hips to the starting position. This is one rep.

Tips and techniques:
• Tighten your buttocks before lifting your hips.
• Keep your hips even and spine neutral as you pull each knee toward your chest.
• Breathe comfortably.

6 | Level 1: Ball squeeze

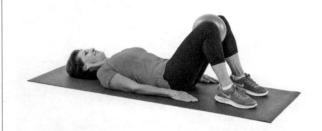

Reps: 8–10
Sets: 1–2
Tempo: 2-2-2
Rest: 30–90 seconds between sets

Starting position: Lie on your back with your knees bent and feet flat on the floor. Put a small ball (roughly 12 inches, or the size of a child's playground ball) between your knees. Place your arms at your sides.

Movement: Tighten your abdominal muscles. Squeeze your knees together against the ball. Hold, then release. This is one rep.

Tips and techniques:
• Exhale as you squeeze, inhale as you release.
• Keep your spine neutral.
• Breathe comfortably.

Level 2: Side-lying inner thigh leg raise

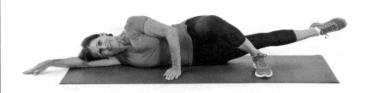

Reps: 8–10
Sets: 1–2
Tempo: 2-2
Rest: 30–90 seconds between sets

Starting position: Lie on your right side with your right leg extended and your head resting on your extended right arm. Bend your left leg at the knee and put your left foot on the floor in front of your right thigh. Place your left hand on the floor at your waistline.

Movement: Tighten your abdominal muscles. Exhale as you lift your right leg up toward the ceiling. Slowly lower your leg to the starting position. This is one rep. Finish all reps, then repeat on the left side. This completes one set.

Tips and techniques:
• Keep your spine neutral.
• Contract your inner thigh as you lift your leg.
• Exhale as you lift, inhale as you lower.

7 | Level 1: Modified side plank

Reps: 2–4 per side
Sets: 1
Tempo: 2-2-2

Starting position: Lie on your right side with your legs extended. Rest your head on your right arm and place your left hand on the floor at your waistline. Align your shoulders and hips evenly. Keep your spine neutral.

Movement: Tighten your abdominal muscles. Exhale as you lift your feet off the floor, keeping your shoulders and hips in a straight line. Hold. Return to the starting position to a count of two. This is one rep. Finish all reps, then repeat on the left side. This completes one set.

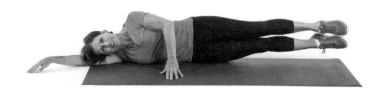

Tips and techniques:
- Keep your head and spine neutral, and your shoulders down and back.
- Focus on squeezing your inner thighs as you lift your feet off the floor.
- Breathe comfortably.

Level 2: Side plank with bent knees

Reps: 1 per side
Sets: 1
Hold: 15–60 seconds

Starting position: Lie on your right side with your knees bent and your feet behind you, stacking your left foot on top of your right foot. Place your left hand on your left hip.

Movement: Tighten your abdominal muscles. Raise your upper body onto your right forearm so that your shoulder is aligned directly over your elbow. While balancing on your right forearm, lift your hips up off the floor, keeping shoulders, hips, and knees in a straight line. Hold. This is one rep. Repeat on your left side. This completes one set.

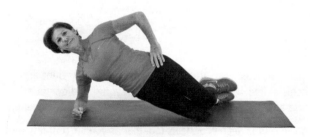

Tips and techniques:
- Keep your head and spine neutral, and align your shoulder over your elbow.
- Breathe comfortably.
- Keep your shoulders down and back.

8 Level 1: Side-lying leg lift

Reps: 8–10
Sets: 1–2
Tempo: 2-2
Rest: 30–90 seconds between sets

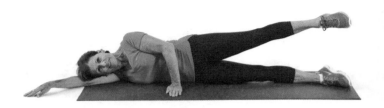

Starting position: Lie on your right side with both legs extended and your head resting on your extended right arm. Place your left hand on the floor in front of your waistline. Align your shoulders and hips evenly, and keep your spine neutral.

Movement: Tighten your abdominal muscles. Raise your left leg toward the ceiling keeping your hips stacked and facing forward. Return to the starting position. This is one rep. Finish all reps before repeating on the opposite side. This completes one set.

Tips and techniques:
• Keep your head and spine neutral.
• Keep your shoulders and hips stacked.
• Breathe comfortably, exhaling as you lift.

Level 2: Clam

Reps: 8–10   **Rest:** 30–90 seconds
Sets: 1–2   between sets
Tempo: 2-2

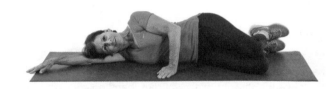

Starting position: Lie on your right side, knees bent and heels in line with your buttocks. Rest your head on your right arm and place your left hand on the floor at your waistline.

Movement: Keep your heels together as you lift your left knee up toward the ceiling as high as is comfortable, then return to the starting position. This is one rep. Finish all reps before repeating on the opposite side. This completes one set.

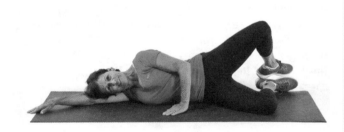

Tips and techniques:
• Keep your hips stacked and still during the movement.
• Lift the top knee up as high as possible without letting the top hip move backward.
• Exhale as you lift.

9 | Level 1: Seated knee extension

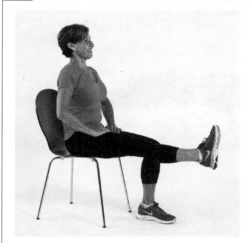

Reps: 8–10
Sets: 1–2
Tempo: 2-2
Rest: 30–90 seconds between sets

Starting position: Sit straight up in a chair with your hands resting on your legs and your feet flat on the floor.

Movement: Exhale as you slowly lift your right foot up toward the ceiling as high as is comfortable, then return to starting position. This is one rep. Finish all reps before repeating on the opposite side. This completes one set.

Tips and techniques:
• Keep your spine neutral and your shoulders down and back.
• Contract your thigh muscles before you lift your foot off the ground.
• Exhale as you lift, inhale as you lower to floor.

Level 2: Single leg raise

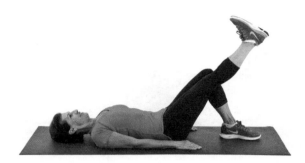

Reps: 8–10
Sets: 1–2
Tempo: 2-2
Rest: 30–90 seconds between sets

Starting position: Lie on your back with your left knee bent, foot flat on the floor, and your right leg extended. Place your hands at your sides.

Movement: Tighten your abdominal muscles. Keeping your right leg straight and foot flexed, lift your foot up toward the ceiling to the height of your bent knee. Return to the starting position. This is one rep. Finish all reps before repeating on the opposite side. This completes one set.

Tips and techniques:
• Flex your foot and tighten the quadriceps muscle on the front of your thigh before you lift your extended leg.
• Keep your spine neutral.
• Breathe comfortably, exhaling as you lift.

10 | Level 1: Front plank on knees

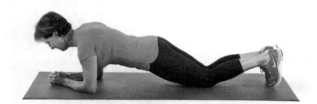

Reps: 1
Sets: 1
Hold: 15–60 seconds

Starting position: Kneel on all fours with your hands and knees directly aligned under your shoulders and hips.

Movement: Tighten your abdominal muscles, and lower your upper body onto your forearms, clasping your hands and aligning your shoulders directly over your elbows. Extend both legs with your feet flexed and toes touching the floor so that you balance your body in a line like a plank. Drop both knees to the floor. Hold. This is one rep.

Tips and techniques:
• Keep your neck and spine neutral during the plank.
• Keep your shoulders down and back.
• Breathe comfortably.

Level 2: Front plank

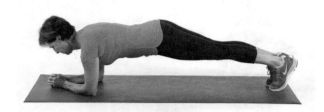

Reps: 2–4
Sets: 1
Hold: 15–60 seconds
Rest: 30–60 seconds between reps

Starting position: Start on your hands and knees.

Movement: Tighten your abdominal muscles and lower your upper body onto your forearms, clasping your hands together and aligning your shoulders directly over your elbows. Extend both legs with your feet flexed and toes touching the floor so that you balance your body in a line like a plank. Hold.

Tips and techniques:
• Keep your neck and spine neutral during the plank.
• Keep your shoulders down and back.
• Breathe comfortably.

Catch your balance: Heel raise

Strictly speaking, the heel raise exercise can't be considered a core exercise because it focuses on strengthening muscles in your calves and ankles. But because these muscles enhance your ability to balance, we're including it as an extra. Core exercises in general strengthen several groups of muscles that stabilize your body, allowing you to remain balanced whether standing stock-still or moving swiftly. The better you can balance, the less likely you are to take a spill if you're walking on uneven ground or unexpectedly stub a toe and stumble. That can add up to fewer bruises and fractures, particularly as you grow older and your bones become more brittle.

Try to do heel raises several times a week. They're easy to fit in while waiting in line (or if that's too embarrassing, try it while talking on the phone). Tai chi and yoga are excellent activities for improving balance, too.

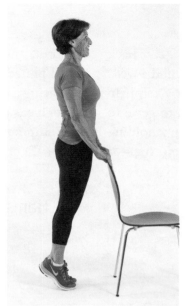

Reps: 8–10   **Rest:** 30–90 seconds
Sets: 1–2   between sets
Tempo: 2-2

Starting position: Stand up straight behind a chair, holding the back of it with both hands. Position your feet hip-width apart and evenly distribute your weight on both feet.

Movement: Tighten your abdominal muscles. Lift up on your toes, letting your heels rise off the floor until you're standing on the balls of your feet. Try to balance evenly without allowing your ankles to roll inward or outward. Lower your heels to the floor, maintaining good posture as you do. This is one rep.

Tips and techniques:

• Zip up and in with your abs. Contract your buttocks, squeezing your inner thighs, and balance on the balls of your feet.

• Imagine you have a string at the top of your head pulling you up. ◗

Home Stretch

Performed on a mat, these six stretches help ease back pain and stiff muscles, while helping you build a well-balanced, flexible core. Stretching regularly can help you feel good all over. If you find it hard to get into the hamstring stretch or pretzel stretch, try holding the ends of a yoga strap placed behind your leg—or substitute the seated hamstring stretch (page 22) or seated pretzel stretch (page 23). For the child's pose, try placing a pillow or rolled towel behind your knees; for cobbler's pose, try a pillow under each knee.

Equipment needed: Exercise mat, yoga strap (optional), pillow or rolled towel (optional).

1 Child's pose

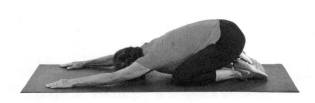

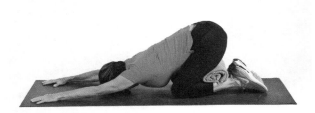

Reps: 2
Sets: 1
Hold: 10–30 seconds

Starting position: Kneel on all fours with knees hip-width apart and feet together.

Movement: Slowly drop your buttocks back toward your heels, extending your arms as far forward as is comfortable. Hold. Return to the starting position. This is one rep.

Tips and techniques:
• Stretch to the point of mild tension, not pain.
• Breathe comfortably.
• If this stretch bothers your knees, place a pillow between your calves and buttocks (see photo).

2 Hamstring stretch lying down

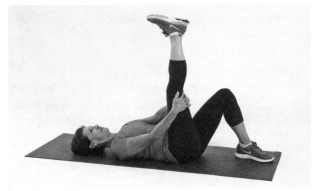

Reps: 2
Sets: 1
Hold: 10–30 seconds

Starting position: Lie on your back with your knees bent and feet flat on the floor.

Movement: Grasp your right leg with both hands behind the thigh. If this is too hard, place a yoga strap or small towel behind your right thigh and hold the ends. Now extend your right leg to lift your right foot toward the ceiling. Straighten the leg as much as possible without locking the knee and flex the ankle to stretch the calf muscles. Hold. Return to the starting position, then repeat with your left leg. This is one rep.

Tips and techniques:
• Stretch to the point of mild tension, not pain. You should feel no pressure behind the knee.
• Keep your shoulders down and back, relaxing them against the floor.
• Breathe comfortably.

3   Pretzel stretch lying down

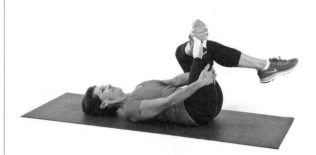

Reps: 2
Sets: 1
Hold: 10–30 seconds

Starting position: Lie on your back with your right knee bent and foot on the floor. Rest your left ankle on your right kneecap. Your left knee should point toward the wall. Grasp the back of your right thigh with both hands. If this is too hard, put a strap or small towel around the back of your right thigh and hold the ends.

Movement: Keep your shoulders down and back, relaxing them against the floor. Slowly lift your right foot off the floor until you feel the stretch in your left hip and buttock. Hold. Return to the starting position. Repeat with your left knee bent and your right ankle resting on your left kneecap. This is one rep.

Tips and techniques:
• Stretch to the point of mild tension, not pain.
• Hold the stretch as still as possible without bouncing.
• Breathe comfortably.

4   Torso rotation stretch lying down

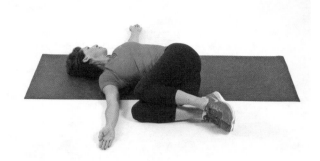

Reps: 2
Sets: 1
Hold: 10–30 seconds

Starting position: Lie on your back with knees bent and feet together, flat on the floor. Put your arms comfortably out to each side just below shoulder level, palms up.

Movement: Tighten your abdominal muscles as you lower both knees together to the right side on the floor. Keeping your shoulders relaxed and pressed against the floor, look in the opposite direction. Feel the stretch across your chest and torso. Hold. Return to the starting position, then repeat in the opposite direction. This is one rep.

Tips and techniques:
• Stretch to the point of mild tension, not pain.
• Try to bring both knees up into the fetal position, or as high as is comfortable.
• Breathe comfortably.

5 Cobbler's pose stretch

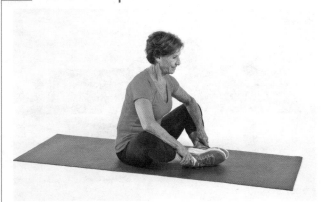

Reps: 2
Sets: 1
Hold: 10–30 seconds

Starting position: Sit on the floor. Bring the soles of your feet together and let your knees fall apart toward the floor.

Movement: Place your hands on your ankles. Hinge forward from your hips until you feel the stretch in your inner thighs. Hold. Return to the starting position. This is one rep.

Tips and techniques:
• Stretch to the point of mild tension.
• Keep your head and spine neutral, your shoulders down and back, and your abdominal muscles tightened.
• Breathe comfortably.

6 Kneeling hip flexor stretch

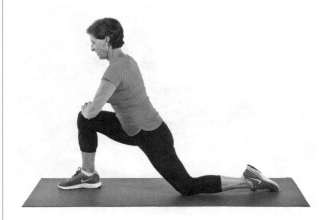

Reps: 2
Sets: 1
Hold: 10–30 seconds

Starting position: Kneel with your hands at your sides.

Movement: Put your right leg in front of you with the knee bent at a 90-degree angle and foot flat on the floor. Place your hands on your right thigh for support. Lean forward, pressing into the hip of your left leg while keeping your right foot on the floor. Hold. Return to the starting position, then repeat with your left leg forward. This is one rep.

Tips and techniques:
• Stretch to the point of mild tension, not pain.
• Keep your head and spine neutral, your shoulders down and back, and your abdominal muscles tightened.
• Breathe comfortably. ▼

Setting goals and motivating yourself

Sticking with exercise isn't always easy. Success is more likely to be yours if you set goals and follow a few tips to boost flagging motivation. If you're spending more time making excuses than doing those planks and bridges, we can help you identify—and smooth out—common bumps in the road.

Choose a goal

Think about it. How will core work benefit you? Check off your goals from the options below, and write a personalized goal in the space provided in "Make your commitment" (page 41) and "My monthly activity calendar" (page 42).

I want to
- ❏ keep my back strong and flexible to help me avoid lower back pain
- ❏ ease back pain or stiffness so I can move, sit, and sleep comfortably
- ❏ enhance my balance and stability, which will help prevent falls while making walking and other activities easier
- ❏ reclaim the strength and flexibility I need for everyday tasks at home like bending, turning, lifting, yanking, reaching items on high shelves, gardening, fix-it work, and housework
- ❏ build up the strength and flexibility I need for on-the-job tasks like lifting heavy items, twisting, or standing or sitting at a desk for hours
- ❏ add power for athletic activities I enjoy like tennis or other racquet sports, a marathon or triathlon, golf, kayaking, and other active pursuits
- ❏ improve my posture, which can trim my figure visually, make clothes fit well, help ease the stress of desk and computer work, and help prevent back injuries
- ❏ help tone my waistline (or use exercise as part of a larger program to slim down)
- ❏ spice up my weekly workouts by adding variation.

Be SMART

Fitting core exercises into your life will pay off in everyday activities, sports successes, a stronger lower back, independent living, and all-around fitness. Sounds great, right? Even so, marshaling the time and will to do these exercises may not be easy. Experts say you're more likely to meet success if you set goals that are **SMART**—that is, specific, measurable, achievable, realistic, and time-based. So as you're setting a goal and penciling it in on the calendar we've provided, make sure it passes the **SMART** test:

S: Set a very **specific** goal. *This week, I will do the "4 excellent exercises for life" on Mondays and Wednesdays.* Or, *I will do a set of front planks on desk plus chair stands on Tuesday, Wednesday, Friday, and Sunday.*

M: Find a way to **measure** progress. *I will log my efforts daily on my calendar, checking off days when I meet my goal.*

A: Make sure it's **achievable**. Be sure you're physically capable of safely accomplishing your goal. If not, aim for a smaller goal initially: *I plan to master four Level 1 exercises, then move on to their Level 2 counterparts.*

R: Make sure it's **realistic**. Choose the change you're most confident you'll be able to make, not the change you most need to make. Focus on sure bets: on a scale of 1 to 10, where 1 equals no confidence and 10 equals 100% certainty, your goal should land in the 7–10 zone. If not, cut it down to a manageable size. For example, *I'll do one front plank on desk three times this week.* Or, *Every week, I'll add five seconds to the length of time I hold front plank on desk.*

T: Set **time** commitments. First, pick a date and time to start. *Starting today, I'll take 10 minutes from my lunch hour to do the Office Workout every Monday, Wednesday, and Friday.* Or, *Starting today, I'll do two stretches after my morning shower, when my muscles are warm, every day for a week.*

Second, choose one weekly check-in time to keep track of whether you're meeting goals or hitting snags. *I'll check my calendar every Friday evening and decide if I should make any changes in my routines to succeed.* Outside deadlines can be really helpful here, too: Signing up for tennis lessons or planning a beach vacation can prod you to get your core program under way.

Motivate yourself

You do your best work when motivated, right? That extends to exercise, too. It's not uncommon to launch a new exercise program raring to go, only to wind up back on the couch with your feet propped up just a few weeks later. If your will wavers, the following tips may help.

■ **Refresh your memory.** Remind yourself how the exercises will help you by reading your goals again (see "Choose a goal," page 39, and "Make your commitment," page 41). Emphasize the positive aspects. Rather than sternly saying, "I *should* do my core exercises," try saying aloud "My back feels better when I do my gentle core exercises and stretches" or "My balance is better when I do my core exercises consistently."

■ **Find the time.** Skimming time from your busy schedule is an art. Here are some ideas that can help. Over the course of a week, skip two half-hour TV shows and use the time to exercise. Fit core exercises into commercial breaks or downtime in your workday. Get up 10 to 15 minutes earlier each day to finish a full workout. Throughout the

Not getting anywhere?

Brainstorming solutions for likely bumps in the road can start you off on the right foot and help keep workouts on track. Once you get going, jot down any hurdles you run into on your monthly activity calendar (page 42) and then think your way around them. Here's some help with common hurdles.

- **Need the okay to start doing core exercises?** Call your doctor today. Remember, it may help to send a copy of the workouts you hope to do, then follow up with a phone call to discuss whether any modifications will be needed.

- **Just don't feel motivated?** Ask a friend to check up on you, or consider working out with a personal trainer or physical therapist, depending on your health issues.

- **Seriously out of shape?** Focus on doing only the easiest exercises over the course of your day. Try our "Easiest abdominal exercises" (see page 18)—maybe just doing one exercise before breakfast, lunch, and dinner every day,

or even every other day, for two weeks. The Office Workout and Office Stretch or Home Stretch are all easy, also.

- **Bored by your routine?** If you've mastered the Level 1 moves, try Level 2 exercises. Done with those? You're ready to step up to our *Core Exercises* Special Health Report, which has six additional core workouts ranging from easy to very challenging. Or add variety by searching online for new core exercises available through reputable fitness organizations, such as the American Council on Exercise fitness library (www.acefitness.org/exerciselibrary).

- **Still stuck?** Sometimes breaking down a bigger goal into smaller steps is the best way to succeed. Instead of aiming for two complete gentle core workouts a week, maybe you can do just one exercise from the "4 excellent exercises for life" (see page 18) and one Home Stretch every day until you cycle through the full set. Then repeat.

day, be on the lookout for pockets of time. Be efficient: As you advance to more challenging exercises, leave the simpler ones behind to make the best use of your time.

■ **Sprinkle core activities throughout your day.** Challenge yourself to see how often you can slip in gentle core work. After your morning shower when muscles are pliable is the perfect time for a few Home Stretch options, such as child's pose and cobbler's pose. While on the phone, do 10 soccer kicks and 10 standing side leg lifts. Before shifting from calls to other projects or back again, do a front plank on desk. If you're not working in an office, take five minutes before lunch to do the bridge, ball squeeze, and heel raise.

■ **Choose cues to serve as a trigger.** While waiting for the light to change, for example, check your posture and practice bracing yourself (see "10 tips for doing gentle core work safely and effectively," page 10). Instead of sipping coffee when your computer is firing up, try a few alternating knee lifts. When you finish a task, take an active break to do side leg lifts or reverse lunges.

■ **Plan simple rewards.** Give yourself a pat on the back for every small or big step toward success. Blast your favorite tune at the end of a workout. Download the "Attaboy" app for your iPhone or iPod

to enjoy a stream of compliments whenever you need to hear it. A bigger reward for staying on track toward your goal for two to four weeks might be new workout gear or sports equipment you'll enjoy.

■ **Get a workout buddy.** Exercising with a friend or family member is more fun, plus you're less likely to cancel on the spur of the moment. If you belong to a gym, ask if there is a buddy program. Or try working out online with a friend via Skype. If finding a real-time or virtual workout buddy isn't possible, go low-tech: ask a friend to check in with you regularly—on workout days or maybe just once a week—to give you a pat on the back or a pep talk.

■ **Reach for your smartphone.** Or iPad, computer mouse, or game system remote. Smartphone fitness apps, health-driven websites, and a slew of fitness games on systems like Wii and Xbox make it easy to set baselines and log calories and activities. Cyber options like these also can help you learn new exercises, track progress, and get friendly nudges that encourage you stick to your goals. Check smartphone fitness options at Apple's app store, Google's Play Store, or Blackberry's App World. Alternately, search the fitness library of the American Council on Exercise (www.acefitness.org/exerciselibrary).

Make your commitment

Now, put your SMART goal and plans together. Start by writing a commitment statement (below). Then fill in "My monthly activity calendar" (see page 42) writing in the times and days you'll do core work, plus any rewards you will give yourself. Here's an example of a commitment statement:

I'm making a commitment to my health, well-being, and enjoyment of life. My goal is to get into better shape and prevent my back from hurting. I plan to start on Wednesday, Jan. 15, by doing the "4 excellent exercises for life" on Wednesdays at 6:30 a.m. and Sundays at 5 p.m. I'll check my calendar weekly on Sunday nights to see if I'm succeeding. If not, I'll brainstorm ways to jump hurdles and motivate myself to get back on track.

Now you try
I'm making a commitment to my health, well-being, and enjoyment of life. My goal is

_____.
I plan to start on _____
by doing _____
on _____.
I'll check my calendar weekly on
_____ to see if I'm succeeding.
If not, I'll brainstorm ways to jump hurdles and motivate myself to get back on track. ♥

My monthly activity calendar

Make copies of the blank calendar below so that you'll be able to fill it out each month. Put each month's calendar in an easy-to-see spot. Then follow these instructions:

→ Month _____

1. Use the notes to the right to jot down your commitment and your reward.

2. Pencil in days and times you plan to do core work, and what you'll be doing (for example, bursts of exercise or a particular workout). Remember, core work should be part of a larger exercise plan, as explained in "How should core work fit into your overall exercise plans?" on page 12. So, when you pencil in your core exercise schedule, it makes sense for you

SUNDAY	MONDAY	TUESDAY	WEDNESDAY

to write down other strength sessions and aerobic activities, too.

3. Put a big splashy check mark next to each success. Anytime you fall short, record the hurdle in the notes section, then try to brainstorm and jot down a solution (see "Not getting anywhere?" on page 40).

4. Once a week, look over what you've checked off. Think about what's working well for you. Decide whether your solutions for jumping hurdles are working, or whether you need to break your goal down into smaller steps in order to be successful (see "Not getting anywhere?" on page 40). And collect any reward due, as planned.

THURSDAY	FRIDAY	SATURDAY

MY COMMITMENT

HURDLES

SOLUTIONS

REWARDS

Resources

Organizations

American Academy of Physical Medicine and Rehabilitation
9700 W. Bryn Mawr Ave., Suite 200
Rosemont, IL 60018
847-737-6000
www.aapmr.org

This professional organization for physiatrists—medical doctors trained in physical medicine and rehabilitation—promotes education. A referral service on the website locates physiatrists by state.

American College of Sports Medicine
401 W. Michigan St.
Indianapolis, IN 46202
317-637-9200
www.acsm.org

ACSM educates and certifies fitness professionals, such as personal trainers, and funds research on exercise. A referral service on the website locates ACSM-certified personal trainers.

American Council on Exercise
4851 Paramount Drive
San Diego, CA 92123
888-825-3636 (toll-free)
www.acefitness.org

ACE is a nonprofit organization that promotes fitness and offers educational materials for consumers and professionals. The ACE website has a referral service to help locate ACE-certified personal trainers and a free video library of exercises.

Institute of Lifestyle Medicine
Joslin Diabetes Center
1 Joslin Place
Boston, MA 02215
617-309-2435
www.instituteoflifestylemedicine.org

Led by Dr. Edward M. Phillips, the medical editor of this report, the Institute is a nonprofit professional education, research, and advocacy organization that is leading a comprehensive effort to reduce lifestyle-related death and disease in society through clinician-directed interventions with patients.

Harvard Special Health Reports

If you've found *Gentle Core Exercises* helpful—or if you're ready to try a more challenging core routine—these four exercise titles from Harvard Medical School can provide additional help. Order them online at www.health.harvard.edu or call 877-649-9457 (toll-free).

Better Balance: Easy Exercises to Improve Stability and Prevent Falls
Suzanne Salamon, M.D., and Brad Manor, Ph.D., Medical Editors
Josie Gardiner and Joy Prouty, Master Trainers
(Harvard Medical School, 2012)

This report explains health problems that may impair balance and prompt falls. The six complete workouts are designed to strengthen muscles, boost confidence, and interrupt a downward spiral that can compromise independence. Checklists help you take steps to ensure personal safety and eliminate home hazards.

Core Exercises: Six Workouts to Tighten Your Abs, Strengthen Your Back, and Improve Balance
Edward M. Phillips, M.D., Medical Editor
Josie Gardiner and Joy Prouty, Master Trainers
(Harvard Medical School, 2013)

The natural next step after mastering the workouts in *Gentle Core Exercises*, the basic *Core Exercises* report offers six additional core workouts with exercises that range from easy to quite challenging. Two workouts call for no equipment other than body weight, while the rest center on exercises done with a medicine ball, stability ball, or Bosu. All exercises can be tailored to make them easier or harder to do.

The Joint Pain Relief Workout: Healing Exercises for Your Shoulders, Hips, Knees, and Ankles
Edward M. Phillips, M.D., Medical Editor
Josie Gardiner and Joy Prouty, Master Trainers
(Harvard Medical School, 2012)

The exercises in this report can help tame ankle, knee, hip, or shoulder pain. When practiced regularly, the workouts may permit people to postpone—or even avoid—joint surgery by strengthening supportive muscles and restoring flexibility.

Strength and Power Training: A Guide for Older Adults
Julie K. Silver, M.D., Medical Editor
(Harvard Medical School, 2013)

Weak muscles hasten the loss of independence as everyday activities become more difficult. Two weekly strength training workouts can help fortify muscles and bones, recouping losses linked to aging or inactivity.